A Hope for ALZHEIMER'S

Hugh Gilbert

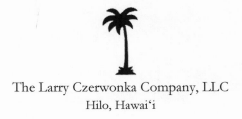

The Larry Czerwonka Company, LLC
Hilo, Hawai‘i

First Edition — June 2014

Published by: The Larry Czerwonka Company, LLC
http://thelarryczerwonkacompany.com

Printed in the United States of America

ISBN: 0692227199
ISBN-13: 978-0692227190

In Loving Memory of my father,
Leo Howard Gilbert 1920 to 2011
an Officer and a Gentleman.

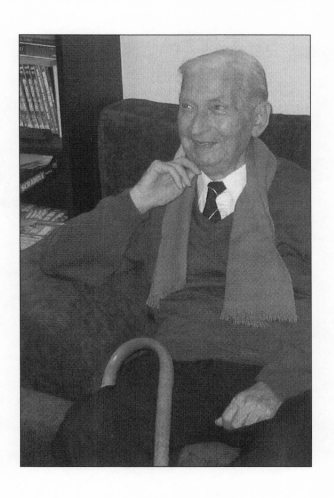

Books by Hugh Gilbert

THE EARLY-AGING WORK FORCE
FREE THE UNICORN

Contents

Contents

Contents

Contents

Contents

Contents

Preface

"The Long Goodbye" is what Alzheimer's disease is now known as internationally. Only those families who are currently living this nightmare with a loved one, or who have gone through it in the past can even begin to comprehend the truly terrifying meaning of this name and the crushing stress and suffering involved for all of the family as the nightmare unfolds. To give some basic perspectives as to the impact this terrible illness has, with as yet no cure or hope of slowing it's progress (until this book) even vaguely in sight, I give you a small sampling of financial ramifications to society.

1. According to the National Audit Office in 2007: "Dementia costs the U.K. economy 20 BILLION pounds per year ($38 Billion Dollars). The costs per person are higher than for all other mental health conditions."

2. According to the U.K. Alzheimer's Society in 2009 in a document called "Counting the Cost"; "Up to 1 in 4 hospital beds at any one time is occupied by a person over the age of 65 who has dementia."

3. According to the U.K. Department of Health in 2009: "By 2039 there will be 1,400,000 people with dementia in the U.K."

We can only shudder at the thought of what those numbers will be in North America and other Continents.

In this book I will offer you some simple, easily defensible strategies, with early intervention being a prime, but not total focus, which, if implemented, could save a minimum of 5% of these costs, the equivalent of a BILLION pounds, or 1.6 BILLION dollars per annum.

Far more importantly and joyfully, we can quantifiably delay the early progression of the condition; improve the quality of life of those suffering and provide their families with at the least, more quality time with their loved ones or, at best, stunning, heart-warming and sustainable improvements in physical capabilities and communication!

The strategies are based on my experiences when dealing with this progressive illness in my father, Leo Gilbert, and are not born of conjecture of any kind. My hope is that many will gain hope and take action in implementing the tools offered, and that enough of a groundswell of public demand will get the attention of the medical community and full University Research Studies will be implemented to prove the validity of my findings. I feel it is worth reemphasising here that the simple strategies that worked for my Dad will have maximum benefit if applied to patients MUCH earlier in the onset of the illness. Time is of the essence.

The first few chapters are difficult to write and possibly to read, however it is vital to have them as it clearly describes the slippery slope of bewilderment and increasing devastation that hundreds of thousands of families have faced and are facing today. Once we get to the point where there seems to be no hope left is when the story shifts as the miracles occurred. Only by realizing just how far down the rabbit hole of Alzheimer's we had gone can you begin to appreciate how wonderful it felt to have stopped the slide and actually have achieved the impossible and be climbing back out towards recovery!

Acknowledgements

My mum, Cathy, who, in her mid-eighties, and trying to recover from bowel cancer surgery and also the loss of vision in one eye, devastated at watching the long goodbye to her husband of over 60 years, kept her tears for many a long lonely night and stood strong for her children and grandchildren as well as being there for my Dad almost every day until the end.

My wife Jane, who fitted in so easily to our family. You were the rock for us all throughout these years, taking care of Mum and Dad in so many ways while keeping me sane in times that often felt like total insanity. My Dad loved you dearly, as do I.

Diana Buchanan, social worker and friend. You gave us direction so many times when we were in shock and lost. Your compassion for humanity was clearly demonstrated consistently as you went far beyond job requirements for us so often and so unselfishly. We would not have made it through without your wisdom and support.

Richard Swift, a true friend and ally who often helped me to re-strategize my efforts and hold laser like focus on the outcomes I was determined to accomplish.

My brothers Howard and John. You both provided unwavering support for Mum and Dad at every step of the way and were always there for me when I faltered.

Debbie, Manager at the care home where my Dad was placed. You believed me right from the start and did everything you could to help us get acceptance from the medical community and your support staff. You gave us hope and support as we took on the medical establishment on so many levels.

The Nursing and support staff at the care home—too many to mention individually. These people showed the highest level of compassion and commitment to everything we tried to do and are frequently denied the praise due to them for doing an amazing job in extremely trying circumstances.

John and Shiela Freil and family, close friends of my parents for 30 years. I could always rely on them to be there for my parents when needed. If, while in my International work commitments, I became concerned as to how things were with my folks, I only had to call them and they would, unreservedly, drop whatever they were doing and drive over to check on them, then give me a call back. This alone made my folks (and my) experience, feel a lot more tolerable. I wish every family was blessed with friends such as these.

My Dad, Leo Howard Gilbert, 1920 *to* 2011. Your quiet courage facing the indignities, vulgarities and outrages of Alzheimer's was constant and exemplary. You faced it all with such a deep and amazing inner strength. May your story be inspirational for many and may it play a role in the ultimate delivery of mankind from the curse of Alzheimer's disease.

Part 1

This is a story of miracles and celebration, not just for my father and his family, but potentially for millions of other Alzheimer's sufferers and their families. The struggle faced by families in coming to terms with the stark reality of the effect of Alzheimer's and the numbing ripple effects which resonate in all directions is an area which has not been adequately addressed on any level. There is little or no professional help available to counsel family members through this protracted nightmare. For the most part we are left to flounder along, with each one of us dealing with it from his or her own personal perspective. It is an unsupportive and helpless environment with no hope for anything other than the certainty of a protracted physically, emotionally and often financially devastating terminal journey. This has to change in the future. However, in my efforts to come to terms with all of this I suddenly became aware of a very bright ray of hope for a potential cure and I was met with resistance on every level as I tried to get my father the chance he so desperately needed. How can a potential cure be simple and easily implemented? Your understandable current doubt and skepticism will gradually dissolve and you will be amazed at the potential of it all.

Chapter 1

The story you are about to read of the last two and a half years of my father's life has apparently become a glowing beacon for many people. I have been told it has been the focus of study groups internationally and is being quoted by families in Hawai'i, North America, South America and Europe as they fight for their loved ones facing similar circumstances. I trust it proves a source of inspiration and understanding for you also.

My father was a strong, highly intelligent, articulate, athletic man who, after a distinguished career in the Royal Navy and Civil Service; worked in positions of trust well into his eighties; and rarely had a sick day in his life. He still spent much time tending to the affairs and not inconsiderable day to day voluntary running of the Stella Maris Organisation in Glasgow, Scotland.

He still lived at home independently with my Mum, his childhood sweetheart and wife for over 60 years and they led a full and dignified life with a huge circle of friends and family.

The fact that each year they would receive over 150 Christmas cards was a testament to the love and esteem they were held in within their community and beyond.

In 2005 (at age 85) he went into hospital for minor prostate surgery and while there he suddenly and shockingly contracted the "superbug" MRSA, which literally almost killed him within days (more on this later), however, despite the high incidence of fatalities from this, he found the inner strength to survive and to some extent recover. It was during the following few years that our family realized that all had not been well at work for Dad. It eventually became clear that he had not been working with full mental acuity for some time, in as much as mistakes and forgetfulness had been becoming more and more prevalent, but as he had no direct supervisor, we all (including Dad) were mostly unaware of how bad things were becoming. He, like most, became adept at keeping conversations to topics he could still relate to so unless you were unusually observant you would have thought he was as sharp as ever.

So, following the MRSA episode, Dad came home from the hospital and his physical recovery continued although mentally there were gradually increasing signs of forgetfulness and occasionally confusion. He still had a sharp intellect and an equally sharp sense of humour, however there were signs of his mental deterioration that were becoming harder to ignore, no matter how we tried to pretend otherwise.

The walls came tumbling down. The illness finally revealed itself, and the effects on other family members gradually, though sometimes suddenly became evident and the devastating collateral damage of Alzheimer's manifested itself. How will you cope should the situation arise in your family?

There is little or no REAL help available to families trying to come to terms with the massive stresses of coping with the advent of Alzheimer's into their world, yet quietly living with the hardest feeling of all. That is the growing fear, emptiness and helplessness of fighting the inevitable tide of impending loss that gnaws silently and unspoken within, until it bursts forth in broken health in others. I am certain that the events that unfolded next are not uncommon scenarios for many.

The stress of coping with Dad's forgetfulness and ever increasing dependence upon her was building up on my Mum more than we realized. Dad had become increasingly possessive, asking where she went, who she was talking to on the phone, why she had to go out etc. (all normal signs of growing dementia and are no reflection on my Dad). She was also going 20 miles by public transport, two or three times per week, to help her almost housebound older brother cope with life as a recent widower, plus go almost daily locally to her younger sister, who lived alone nearby and was coping with progressive terminal illness. So, besides bringing groceries to them and dealing with Dad, Mum really didn't have a lot of time for herself anymore. She had been a very social individual, a founder member of her church choir and loved not only to sing, but also the buzz of social interactions with her friends there. Gradually this social life had eroded until it was non-existent. She never complained and focused on her husband, brother and sister completely and unselfishly. Many a time shedding quiet tears as Dad lay sleeping beside her, she prayed for the strength to get through the next day and to keep the growing severity of the problem away from her sons and their families.

The stress on my Mum took its inevitable toll. While trying to cope and also prepare for the upcoming Christmas Season she became aware that something was not right with her own health and decided not to worry anyone and try to carry on as before. Finally her symptoms became so persistent that she saw her physician and, after going for further tests, she was unable to protect us any longer. The tests confirmed a malignancy in her bowel, requiring urgent surgery. She was told her chances of survival were questionable and that she would need to have the added insult to her dignity of a stoma (a bag attached to her abdomen) for the foreseeable future afterwards.

Suggestion #1

"You have an obligation to protect the caregiver (in this case my Mum) just as much as to protect and support the loved one suffering from Alzheimer's."

The one who is caring for the other is on a slippery slope to a breakdown in their health as well. They are caring for a loved one in often almost intolerable circumstances as the dementia increases. The constant worry and stress of dealing with the complete unpredictability of their loved ones behaviour takes an unavoidable toll. Do NOT listen to them when they stoically tell you that they are coping well. Either step in to help them yourself or get professional assistance involved in day to day care immediately. In retrospect I wish we had taken this step a long time before the end game kicked off.

Note: I have witnessed several families (thankfully not mine) where some of the grown children do not recognize the toll being exacted on the caregiving partner and have watched these partners deteriorate rapidly and often do not outlive their spouse! If you do not recognize and own the obligation to protect them, then the chances are high that you may be facing the impending loss of more than one family member!

(To further compound our scenario . . . on the same day, while Mum was being told the diagnosis, unknown to her, her younger sister [my aunt and godmother]who had suffered mightily yet stoically, was being admitted into the Palliative Care unit of the nearby General Hospital and was given a short time to live.)

In shock, Mum returned home from hearing her own diagnosis, supported by her niece, and tried to tell Dad as gently as possible of what lay ahead. Although often confused, the impact of their words hit hard, he did not speak a word and within a few hours was experiencing a heart attack and was rushed into hospital, and admitted to a ward within meters of my Mum's sister!

Dad's cardiac symptoms settled over 48 hours yet physically and mentally he deteriorated rapidly in that ward and had changed within days from the image of a sharply dressed and mostly coherent individual to a seriously ill and physically weak man, wearing only a pyjamas and slippers, frequently incontinent of urine (or so it seemed), barely able to walk more than a few meters, and at times, having difficulty conversing sensibly with us. My wife, Jane would take his pyjamas home each night and wash and iron them without letting my brothers see, so that they would not be alarmed by his apparent incontinence.

I now put the prime reason for his rapid deterioration firmly on dehydration, and his apparent incontinence on high demands placed on inadequate numbers of staff in his ward, and will give my solid reasons for feeling this way later in this story.

There is beauty in every scenario in life however and it was a joy to us all to see his face light up with happiness each time my Mum came to visit him, which usually was twice daily. He even knew her footsteps coming down the hallway and would be beaming at her as she entered the ward.

Even to the very end he always seemed to sense her energy and would glow with happiness in her presence.

Once again my mother gathered her strength and held her head high as she ministered to her sister, to her brother and to my Dad, while making arrangements for her own surgery. She would not schedule it until she had helped her sister to pass, which somewhat mercifully happened within weeks and she scheduled herself to be admitted to hospital for her surgery literally within 2 hours of overseeing that her younger sister's funeral wishes had been honoured and fully implemented!

My Dad, while confused, somehow, in his lucid moments, clearly remained aware of the other traumas unfolding around him, and, true to character, tried to be of as little a burden as possible and kept his thoughts and fears to himself.

We did, with careful planning, manage to bring him home for a few hours on Christmas Day and he happily shared a Christmas dinner with us all as we all wondered what the near future would hold.

We as a family were now suddenly faced with the prospect of not only losing my Dad, but, due to the severity of Mum's diagnosis plus her physical and emotional exhaustion were also facing the unspoken possibility of losing them both. The walls of perceived family invincibility were indeed crashing down around us now.

Chapter 3

Mum was admitted to hospital within hours of her sister's funeral . . . and her surgery was scheduled for the next morning. We first took her up to the ward where my Dad was, so they could say their hopefully temporary farewell to each other. They both stoically supported each other and it was clear that Dad understood what was about to transpire. Mum was then admitted to pre-surgery and somehow kept an amazing facade of calmness to us as we sat with her that evening (actually, on reflection we all kept the façade of composure going, as families do in these times). Her surgery the next day took several hours and the first good news we had was that she had survived the operation, and would be in the High Dependency Unit (ICU) for a few days. By the third day she had stabilized and we took Dad over in a wheelchair to visit her briefly, so they could see each other again. That was a wonderful moment for us all, most of all for them as they both wept quiet tears of joy.

Now we could begin to plan to get Mum home again and begin her recovery. Dad was being well cared for in the hospital (or so we thought) so would be ok for a while till we got Mum back on her feet, then decisions on the future could be made as appropriate.

Just when we were celebrating Mum's survival and feeling as though we, as a family may have gotten a handle on things, everything exploded around us yet again.

Chapter 4

"Your Father must be placed elsewhere!" those were the words we were told by the ward physician, out of the blue to us and within a week of Mum's surgery!

My dad had suddenly become even more confused, was very weak and was apparently urinary incontinent! The Hospital informed my partner Jane and me that we would have to find alternative accommodation for him as they needed the bed!

Suggestion #2

When you have a relative beginning to show early signs of any form of Dementia, have the foresight to find what care home facilities are available locally for if and when the time should come.

Ask for a full tour of each of them and be clear as to what level of care each provides and what are the admission criteria. Families don't do this because they feel guilty and because they are still in denial that it won't become necessary.

We could have, and on reflection should have, gone around these care homes at least a year prior to being confronted with the necessity. We could have done this without telling or upsetting my mother and thus been much better prepared to deal with it.

Already hit hard by recent events, this latest hammer blow was hard for us to take indeed. We decided not to tell Mum right away as she was still in the acute stages of post op recovery. She had suffered a complication and had nearly lost the sight from one of her eyes!

It was then that we contacted social services for advice and met Dianne Buchanan, a Quarrier Homes social worker extraordinaire, whose unsung work in the community is legend in our eyes.

She explained the admission criteria for care home residency and gave us locations of several, offering such patience and support to us as she guided us along. It was important that we tried to keep Dad in close proximity to his home so Mum could visit him regularly when she got home.

It is a terrible numbness that engulfs family as you visit these care homes for the first time and realise that you are negotiating terms to have your father committed into care. However within days he had been assessed and accepted in principle for two fairly local residences.

Others had been rejected by us completely as we could not believe how depressing and frankly frightening they were. I told my partner that if I ever got to be that in need of care that I would rather travel to Geneva for assisted legal suicide than face confinement in some of these places we had visited.

The fact that Dad was being placed in care caused turmoil within the family as several simply did not understand the gravity or severity of the situation and insisted that he was "not that bad" while others were simply in a state of denial.

The fact was however, that the Hospital had TOLD us to get Dad placed in a care home immediately and it was not something we had any choice around.

I now know that this conflict and confusion is common in families faced with these decisions and understand that everyone copes differently with loss, but at the time it was just another stress to be addressed. Some family members simply cannot come to terms with the reality of the situation their loved one will not be able to cope at home and that they now require 24 hour care.

My Mum would need rest as she recovered from her major surgery, and the hospital was leaving us without an option for Dad.

We told everyone to think of it as a temporary measure, yet in our hearts we knew this most likely would not be the case.

Suggestion #3

Moving Dad created a lot of hurt internally in our family, as I'm sure it has in millions of others. Things were said in the chaos of the moment that left scars for some time to come. On reflection none of it was meant as negative or intended to hurt, but was simply an understandable response to the insanity we were all being forced to deal with. Please, please realise that stress affects each family member differently and they will process their grief differently, and sometimes even wear rose tinted glasses of denial—the first stage of grieving. Do not try to get everyone feeling the same or to take anything they may say personally. It will only create even more pain and stress if you do. Everyone recognise each other's right to be confused and afraid and simply be as compassionate as you can while remembering to be gentle on yourself too!

In the meantime my father had deteriorated rapidly mentally and barely had a sensible conversation with us. However, a vacancy quickly came open in the care home that had been our second choice and he was first on the waiting list to be transferred to our first choice, which was a comparatively bright and cheerful place, must easier for my Mum to come and visit after she had recovered sufficiently.

A couple of days later Dad was transferred to the care home and the next stage of the journey into the abyss of Alzheimer's ready to unfold.

Chapter 5

The care home that Dad was admitted to was an old converted large stone building, formerly a school for local children in post World War II Glasgow.

The staff were very caring and gentle with Dad on admission and certainly seemed more attuned to the needs of the dementia residents than had often been the case in the General Hospital.

This was mostly due to staff shortages in the General Hospital in my opinion and is no reflection on any individual there.

This was somewhat encouraging to us in a way and eased the transition just a little. However I must digress a little here and jump forward a week, for within that week of receiving lots of more personal care and his water intake being increased dramatically and monitored daily my father was up walking around with a walker frame (sometimes only with a cane) and could manage to get to the toilet on his own!

It was clear to us that he had become severely dehydrated while in hospital, which had contributed greatly to his physical weakness and mental confusion and that he had hit the assist button at his bedside for help to get to the toilet but, due to short staffing that staff had not always been able to get to him, resulting in him urinating himself and being diagnosed as incontinent! We were delighted to see him up and around again and, while stunned and angry at the previous care he had received were simply glad that they made us get him out of there as it was patently clear to us that if he had stayed there that he would have been close to death by now!

Suggestion #4

To all readers, if you see a loved one deteriorate rapidly in similar circumstances, please ensure that their fluid intake is closely monitored and that they are being given adequate and timely assistance to reach the toilet when they need it. Please also insist that if they are deteriorating that they may well be dehydrated and could be rehydrated by means of a saline drip intravenously where possible, as recovery of mental alertness due to this simple intervention can often be instant and seemingly miraculous.

Many senior citizens at home are also poorly hydrated, particularly if living alone and this should be closely monitored by family and medical support staff. However, now you know and fully understand what appeared to be the first miracle we witnessed on our family journey together.

Chapter 6

My first stunning insight into a possible cause of, or at least a massive contributory factor in, the onset of dementia/Alzheimer's disease.

Now, return with me in time to the morning of the second day of Dad's admission into the care home. Dad had, it seemed, almost gone into sudden shock over the move from the hospital in such a weak state and seemed much worse to me. He sat by his bedside, dressed only in a hospital gown, looking straight through me with no sign of recognition and had just wet himself, clearly unaware of it happening.

(Remember this was immediately after his transfer, he was in shock and only a few days later would be walking around with a cane again as described in the previous chapter! This is why we referred to it as the first miracle we witnessed.)

The carers compassionately got him cleaned up and lifted him back into his bed, where he quickly drifted off to sleep. I just sat there watching him, happy that he was sleeping peacefully and trying to come to terms with all that had happened to him and to our family in the past few weeks. Dad began to snore, softly at first, then rising to an extremely loud level indeed. I found myself grinning at him as the decibel count rose and I mused that I had never known my Dad snored. I wondered how many other things I didn't know, and may now never know about him.

Then the rhythmical loud snoring changed and he began to hold his breath, sometimes for as long as thirty seconds, before beginning to breathe again with a loud snort! I am a Physical Therapist by profession and immediately recognised this to be what is known as Cheyne-Stokes respiration which is a prime symptom of sleep apnoea.

As I continued to reflect, I wondered how long Dad had had these symptoms. My mother later confirmed that he had slept that way for over 30 years!

I was suddenly startled by the realisation that sleep apnoea is surely a clear indicator of oxygen deprivation to the body, and, more relevant in this case, to the brain!

My questions then surfaced clearly.

Suggestion #5

My Questions regarding sleep apnoea:

"Could this 40 years of nightly O_2 (oxygen) deprivation to the brain be a contributing factor to the aberrant changes in cellular structure and diminishment in size of the brains of dementia/Alzheimer's sufferers?"

If so, then, "Could an increase in that oxygen supply give some return of physical and mental capability and function to my Dad and in fact to the millions of other dementia/Alzheimer's sufferers globally?"

And, beyond that, "If my first question was true, then could oxygen possibly be used as a preventative measure for the millions of others showing early signs of dementia?"

It all made sense to me and I determined in that one shining moment to commit myself completely to a quest for answers. I immediately realised that most of the treatment and research on Alzheimer's causes and cures was focussed on the resolution of the cellular changes in the brain tissue (known as plaques). Well, what if the plaques were forming over time due to prolonged lack of oxygen to the brain? That could indicate the treatment was being aimed at a symptom and not the cause!

I left Dad asleep in his room and headed home, for the first time feeling a distinct flicker of excitement and a ray of hope around the insanity of it all.

Chapter 7

My father clearly showed that extra sensory perceptions
can increase when we have dementia!

While the introduction of increased hydration had made an amazing
difference to Dad in the first few days of being in the care home and
he was no longer incontinent and could walk well with his walker frame
he was still terribly confused. He seemed to recognise us somewhat
now although conversation would wander he could only hold focus on
a thought briefly.

However, I remind you that his placement was in a large old stone
building that had been a school for a large dockside population on
post-war Glasgow. I know for sure that Dad had no concept of the
previous use of the building One day, after about a week there, we
were escorting him back from the day room to go upstairs to his room
when he suddenly stopped in his tracks and would not move. He refused to pass by a particular doorway and resisted any and all efforts to
get him to move. He was clearly upset, saying that he could not and
would not go past that door because "the children are in there!" It was
a full 20 minutes before staff managed to get him into a wheelchair and
calm enough to get him back upstairs in the elevator to his room,
where he settled down peacefully again to sleep.

As far as we know he never mentioned it or had a similar episode
again. I have no doubt that he indeed sensed something strongly
around the children who had been there all those decades previously.
On a personal level, while the staff did their best for the most part, I
had never felt that the energy in the building was comfortable, but had
put that down to my own personal discomfort and difficulty adjusting
to the world of care homes.

Suggestion #6

When your loved ones become agitated do not simply dismiss it as their being delusional, they may well be having an experience beyond our comprehension, and it is just as terrifying for them as it would be for us.

Support them as best you can until they are calm again. It wouldn't hurt to establish if there has been a history of paranormal activity in the building or in their room before.

I know this may sound a little off the wall to some of you, but I can only relate it as it happened and give the best advice accordingly.

So, in the meantime, my mother had been released from the hospital and was home again, weak, almost blind in one eye and suffering the indignity of a colostomy bag, but already was going to see Dad every day. She was delighted to see him so much better physically although quite distressed at the lack of good conversation. She was unaware of just how close Dad had been to death just 5 days earlier in the General Hospital.

On a side note here, my mother was given home help service, whereby she was allowed 4 visits a day if needed to make up to 3 meals a day and assist in getting into bed etc. I seem to recall that these poor workers were so rushed that they only had around 15 minutes per visit, sometimes singly or in pairs (and what kind of nutritional meals can be prepared in 15 minutes?). This was disruptive at first as it was often a different and new caregivers who would call and Mum was not comfortable with so many strangers in her home. This meant that instead of being able to relax that Mum was being taken care of, my wife Jane would often get to her home before the carers got there first thing in the morning. Also, it would appear that some of these wonderful ladies do not have sufficient practical skills for the job. One day my Mum said that all she wanted to eat was a "3 Minute Hard Boiled Egg" . . . the caregiver then took Jane into the kitchen and asked her how long did that mean she had to boil it! We laughed long and hard about that later.

Suggestion #7

If your parent, living at home, eventually requires home care assistance, make certain that a family member is at hand every day for the first few days until your parent becomes comfortable with the individual(s) and the process.

Suddenly Dad deteriorated again rapidly within 3 days and quickly became bedridden and even more incoherent! Thankfully we had learned our lesson and my brother demanded to see Dad's file and noticed that his fluid intake had become minimal. He went ballistic (well done, brother!) and formally complained to care home management. Dad was put on a saline drip and his water intake monitored and he recovered in just three days!

I stress that for the most part the staff and the standard of care had been satisfactory to us, however this should reemphasise the urgency of monitoring fluid intake in these patients. I don't understand why more emphasis is not placed on this as standard practice in ALL care homes (it is in some) and is certainly something you should make sure is in place, before placing a loved one in their care. Also, at least once a week, ask to see their patient file/chart and check on fluid levels being recorded. The fact that you do this consistently seems to make staff more aware of their accountability and, I feel, results in fewer incidents of dehydration.

It was just as Dad made his rapid return to "normal" that we received word that there was now a vacancy in the care home that we had preferred and within a day Dad was transferred there.

Chapter 8

Transition into a brighter world.
We adjust and refocus on Dad's possible recovery!

The new care home dad was now in was in a much newer and brighter facility, with a completely different energetic to the previous building he was in. He was welcomed warmly and settled in quickly to the routines. Mum was now strong enough to visit him every day and she never missed. Thankfully it was much closer for her to get to also. She was now slowly regaining weight and was gathering her own strength to return to the hospital and have the stoma bag removed and the procedure hopefully reversed!

She had been given the welcome news that she was cancer free!

In our eyes another miracle had occurred when we heard this wonderful news.

Now she determined that she did not want to live if it meant the continued indignity of the stoma bag and chose to take her chances on the reversal surgery. She no longer required the home care as such and had returned to making her own meals. Housework was still an issue however so my wife and I arranged for and paid for a home cleaning lady to attend her twice a week. We continued to pay for this, plus her phone bill and TV service for the next two years. When everything is in such chaos it is important that stresses be kept to a minimum for the caregiving spouse, so families should quietly take on some of these financial responsibilities during the time of crisis. It was important also that she had other outlets so we visited her regularly, helped her reestablish normalcy with outward activities such as shopping, seeing friends, going for day trips with us, family dinners, staying overnight in our home etc. She would not stay longer than one night in our home as she was committed to being at Dad's side no matter what may befall her.

Suggestion #8

When a parent is initially placed in a care home facility, often it is the one who has taken care of the finances throughout their marriage. The remaining parent is initially totally bewildered by the apparent complexity of handling ongoing bills etc. and has much worry as to how future income (pensions etc.) will be impacted by their current situation. Therefore it is imperative that family are aware of this and quietly set about taking care of some of the bills by paying for the basics until everything has settled into a routine again. In our case, to ease the transition, as stated, we paid for Mum's phone bill, her Television billings and for 2 years we paid for the carer who eventually was employed to come into her home twice a week for 2 hours each time. Each family should find their own ways of providing such support and discuss it well in advance of the need arising.

This may not be necessary at all but should be prepared for and once implemented can take two to three years before no longer being necessary.

Chapter 9

The journey towards having oxygen accepted as treatment for dementia/
Alzheimer's continued. Feeling lost, and often disheartened, in a
wilderness of ignorance from the system we are asked to trust,
I pressed forward and found my first proof!

Feeling lost, and often disheartened, in a wilderness of ignorance from the system we are asked to trust, I pressed forward.

Armed only with a growing certainty and urgency that oxygen deprivation through sleep apnoea could be a massive factor in the cause of and possibly the recovery from Alzheimer's disease, I tentatively began to discuss this with staff at the new care home and with my own family.

I quickly came to realize that the thought of a resident improving was an utterly foreign concept to staff and management alike, and I struggled deeply with the awareness of the truth that my father had simply been placed into an environment to die. Why then, do they not recognize this truth advertise it as the Palliative Care environment that in truth it is? (And apply for government assistance to provide better service?)

Suggestion #9

When you have a relative in a care home scenario please understand that, to staff there, the thought that a patient in their care may actually improve is almost beyond their comprehension initially. This has never happened to any of their patients in the past and is understandably a completely foreign and illogical concept for them. Be prepared to use this story as a means of education as it will be vital for you to get them on board as quickly as possible. If your loved one is still at home it should be much easier to pursue.

Next, discussing the concept with my family was not simple either. In any family there will be a natural and understandable massive variance in considering anything outside of the *norm*. Some will still be in deep shock and not have come to terms with the fact that their mother/father or spouse is indeed beginning the long goodbye, others will have resigned themselves to it and are unable to open their hearts enough again to an apparently *random* and unheard of proposition of hope. This will be the case in most families and should be understood with compassion.

My first logical step was to approach my father's long time family physician.

On July 1st 2009 I wrote:

Dear Dr. xxxxxxx,

This is Hugh Gilbert, Cathie and Leo's son from Canada.
Jane and I are home in Scotland for 3 months again and doing our best to make sure Mum and Dad are happy.

My question is around my father at this point. When he was at his worst, a few months ago, I was sitting in a chair in his room, watching him sleep and reflecting on all that had transpired.

I gradually became aware of his having sleep apnoea, with Cheyne-Stokes breathing etc., etc. It was quite startling to witness how long he could actually go without breathing!

So, I asked Mum how long he had been this way and she said for as long as she could remember! So, it strikes me that prolonged oxygen deprivation could well be a component of many forms of dementia and I intend to ask the care home at xxxxxxxx as to how many of their patients have Apnoea.

I would like your opinion if you feel that daily oxygen could harm my Dad in any manner, and, if not, I will pay to get it set up and see if there are any measurable results.

There is something else I have been researching but will discuss that with you at a later date.

My Mobile phone # is xxxxxxxxxx
Many Thanks,
Hugh

Then I contacted Alzheimer's Scotland and Alzheimer's U.K.
On July 24th 2009 I wrote both of these organisations:

Dear Sir/Madam,

As one of the many who have a loved one suffering from Alzheimer's disease I have attached a letter which I recently sent to my father's physician complete with my rationale behind it.

How many kinds of dementia have actually been triggered by sustained oxygen deprivation, such as sleep apnoea, over the years?

My thinking has made sense to everyone I have discussed it with both locally and internationally, public and professionals alike.

Please read it, give it your thought and pass it on if appropriate. I would love to hear your thoughts also.

Best Wishes,
Hugh Gilbert

The family physician's response was slow in coming and, when it did, was very resistant to the concept of Oxygen as an intervention, stating that it could be dangerous. Firstly my Dad's Physician said that she had seen no research on this and secondly that Oxygen could be dangerous. The first part of her statement only made me determined to find research, while the second part somewhat stunned me as I have seen Oxygen Bars freely available in airports for years, and Autistic Children, Parkinson's patients and others are often placed in Hyperbaric Chambers for full body *oxygenation* saturation. There are even *designer* oxygen inhalers available in nightclubs in London. Surely a clinical trial of oxygen for my Dad could not hold the same potential dangers as the myriad of increasing medications he was being prescribed (which give no hope of a cure or even of slowing the disease).

My Father was dying day by day and his integrity constantly assaulted. . . . What exactly did we have to lose here? I was simply asking for oxygen!

My father demonstrated none of the standard major contraindications of using oxygen (CHRONIC lung or serious heart issues) so I was forced to look for another entry point for him to use a trial of oxygen. The only positive direction I received from Alzheimer's Scotland and Alzheimer's U.K. was to contact Alzheimer's Europe which I did and after several fruitless communications I eventually got my first ray of hope!

Dear Mr. Gilbert,

Thank you for your email concerning sleep apnoea and sorry for the delay in answering which was due to the fact that I was not in the office. We do not have any information in our database about obstructive sleep apnoea. However, a study was carried out at the University of California, San Diego School of Medicine by Sonia Ancoli-Israel and was published in the November 2008 issue of the Journal of the American Geriatric Society. I attach links to articles which briefly describe this study.

http://bit.ly/treatsnore and also http://bit.ly/treatapnoea

The study looked at the effect of continuous positive airway pressure on cognitive functioning in people with Alzheimer's disease and obstructive sleep apnoea. As you will see, Dr. Sonia Ancoli-Israel is quoted as having said: "Although it is unlikely that OSA causes dementia, the lowered oxygen levels and sleep fragmentation associated with OSA might worsen cognitive function." In the actual article, the authors conclude:

"This study was not an epidemiological study, and the prevalence of OSA in those with mild to moderate AD is uncertain, although the data show there is a nontrivial proportion of patients with AD for whom OSA is a clear problem. It has been suggested that OSA might be a reversible cause of cognitive loss and dementia and that treatment of OSA, especially in the early stages of dementia when patients are still largely independent, may slow dementia progression. The results of this study in which CPAP treatment of OSA improved cognitive function in patients with mild to moderate AD, lend support to that hypothesis. Further studies will need to determine whether CPAP treatment of OSA in patients with AD might slow dementia progression. In the meantime, clinicians who care for patients with AD with OSA need to consider implementing CPAP treatment."

On Monday I will be attending our board meeting and will ask if the board members are aware of any research in their countries into OSA as a possible cause of dementia.

Best regards

Dianne Gove

FINALLY I had the results of a real study supporting my hypothesis as viable, and this was most exciting to read. It truly felt like a prayer had been answered. There was now a very bright chink of light in the darkness. My response was a follows:

Dear Dianne,

Many thanks for your prompt and informative response. I apologise if my frustration was evident in my correspondences, however, it seems I have been met with such indifference at times on many levels as I have fought to have someone consider my hypothesis. My Father is in a Nursing home in Glasgow, Scotland and we are watching him slip away mentally, with the agonising slowness and the uncompassionate relentlessness of Alzheimer's.

I am now aware that he has been exhibiting symptoms of sleep apnoea (Cheyne-Stokes et al.) for well over 30 years, but had never mentioned it to a physician. His Physician says "oxygen can be dangerous" and appears reticent in attempting A) Diagnosis of OSA and then B) Implementation of CPAP.

Your articles give me great hope, tempered with realism, that at least I may be able to find a way to at least try CPAP with him, but I know that in his case that time is of the essence.

For millions of others worldwide in the early stages of dementia, however, there would appear to be a genuine avenue of exploration with CPAP which I am sure they would embrace. Earlier screening into the presence of sleep apnoea as standardised medical investigation may also pre-empt many of the later tragedies which we as a family face today.

Thank you for bringing this forward to your Board Meeting,

 Please keep me advised,

God Bless You,

Hugh Gilbert

I then immediately contacted the author of the article:

Dear Professor Ancoli-Israel,

I have been advised to contact you by the European Alzheimer's Society. I am convinced that Sleep Apnoea, Oxygen Deprivation, plays a pivotal and underestimated role in many cases of dementia.

I have been fighting to find someone who may at least be in partial agreement. I have been dealing with Dianne Gove at Alzheimer's Europe and she has been extremely helpful. I will forward you our most recent correspondences for you to briefly peruse.

While I truly feel this link between apnoea and dementia will soon be recognized and clients can be put on CPAP in the very early stages of exhibiting dementia symptomology, my father is in Nursing Care in Scotland and we are watching him slip away painfully slowly. I/he do not have time for the clinical trials which may take interminably long to complete. How can I get his physician to approve a trial of CPAP to at least say that we tried?

Blessings,

Hugh Gilbert

Her response came October 9th 2009 as follows:

I am sorry to say that I don't know how to get physicians to treat apnoea in this group of patients. I am attaching my research article in case you want to share it with the physician.

Best of luck,

Sonia Ancoli-Israel, Ph.D.

Professor of Psychiatry

Director, Gillin Sleep and Chronomedicine Research Center

Department of Psychiatry

University of San Diego

So now, after three months of trying, at least I finally had an article in hand that PROVED a potential link to improved cognitive function in Alzheimer's patients but was no further forward in getting my father given a simple test to prove he had sleep apnoea!

This article at least began to give my family hope as they realised that there may be some merit in what I had been claiming.

Chapter 10

I uncover even more University Research which provides the ABSOLUTE
PROOF that I have been correct in all of my claims
and in my efforts to get help for my father!

Then a SECOND REPORT was given to me less than one week later
on October 14th 2009! This study not only confirmed the benefits of
oxygen for dementia patients but also sensationally supported and confirmed my claims that:

1. "Some studies show that as many as 70% to 80% of all dementia patients also suffer from sleep apnoea!"

2. "Scientists at The University of San Diego, California, last year
   for the first time showed that treating sleep apnoea in patients
   with Alzheimer's actually seemed to improve cognitive function"

3. "Specifically, putting patients with mild to moderate
   Alzheimer's on a machine that delivers pressurised air into the
   lungs during sleep over the course of six weeks resulted in improved test scores for things like verbal learning and mental
   processing!"

And now the biggest breakthrough of all:

4. "A Study by the University of Washington School of Medicine
   found that chronic sleep deprivation makes the brain plaques
   that characterise Alzheimer's disease appear earlier and more
   often."

This is EXACTLY what I had been claiming since day one!

(This article appeared in the *Red Deer Advocate* newspaper [Red Deer
Alberta, Canada] on Oct. 1st 2009 by Lee Bowman and was discussing a
publication in the medical journal, *Diabetes Care*.)

I hastily combined both research reports, now in my possession, and sent them to all the Alzheimer's Societies, the family physician and every friend I could think of.

This whole chapter will constitute Suggestion #10.

And still the physician had not ordered a simple test for sleep apnoea for my Dad, and he was deteriorating slowly but steadily.

Suggestion #10

This article was published in the *Red Deer Advocate* newspaper(Red Deer, Alberta, Canada) on Oct. 1st 2009 by Lee Bowman and was discussing a publication in the medical journal, Diabetes Care.

This is powerfully important information for families who are trying to get access to oxygen to help their loved ones.

1. "Some studies show that as many as 70% to 80% of all dementia patients also suffer from sleep apnoea!"

2. "Scientists at The University of San Diego, California, last year for the first time showed that treating sleep apnoea in patients with Alzheimer's actually seemed to improve cognitive function"

3. "Specifically, putting patients with mild to moderate Alzheimer's on a machine that delivers pressurised air into the lungs during sleep over the course of six weeks resulted in improved test scores for things like verbal learning and mental processing!"

4. "A Study by the University of Washington School of Medicine found that chronic sleep deprivation makes the brain plaques that characterise Alzheimer's disease appear earlier and more often."

Please pay FULL attention to this last statement. It is compelling evidence of the proof you have been looking for.

Chapter 11

Even after presenting my findings to the physician, Alzheimer's Scotland
and Alzheimer's Europe the medical resistance remained high,
it felt as if I was being sandbagged and stonewalled at every turn.

The care home where my father was became my only hope as they had become very supportive of my efforts. I could sense the excitement in the staff there as they began to consider the possibility that some of the patients in their care may actually have hope of improvement! This had an uplifting effect on THEIR morale coming to work each day.

They had realized that several other care home residents had sleep apnoea also and they were beginning to openly wonder if these patients may also benefit from a trial of oxygen!

Therefore I took the next logical step of asking the Medical Consultant in charge of medical care in the care home if he would approve a medical prescription for oxygen for my father if I could indeed prove that he had sleep apnoea? Two problems arose immediately. Firstly the consultant (who was a psychiatrist) could only consider a request if it came from the family physician. This, as we knew, was not going to happen. Secondly he simply informed me that my father was not a suitable candidate for oxygen! To the best of my knowledge the consultant had never examined my father. I should state at this point that I had many years of experience around oxygen application as I was Senior Therapist in charge of chest and lung care and drainage in High Dependency Units (ICU) and also chronic care wards in General Hospital settings as Director of Physical Therapy department for years in Canada and am well aware of the contraindications for oxygen therapy in a small percentage of the elderly population.

So, there we were, stalled yet again. I had uncovered the research that I had been told did not exist, I was simply asking for a standard test to prove the presence of sleep apnoea, and, if positive, for a trial of standard oxygen treatment to be implemented, yet receiving absolutely no support from any of the Alzheimer's Organisations, and being simply refused any consideration by the family physician or the care home Consultant Physician.

Meanwhile my Dad was still slipping slowly away from us. He was no longer walking, seldom truly recognised anyone except my Mum, did not know what he wanted to eat, could not recognise the clock on the wall or the watch on his wrist, and his speech was mostly rambling and incoherent. We were really beginning to lose hope at this point and were probably at one of the lowest points in the journey.

Chapter 12

I bring in a kit and get my father tested for sleep apnoea and also see if he will tolerate the nasal applicator needed to deliver oxygen into his system.

We finally prove that my father has sleep apnoea and therefore is indeed a candidate for oxygen therapy.

All this time I had been actively trying to find a private company to send me a test kit for my Dad to confirm that he indeed had sleep apnoea. I pressed on, without physician consent, to get the test done privately and had received the go ahead from the care home management to proceed if and when I was ready.

Suggestion #11

The U.K. Company who provided the kit to test my father for a diagnosis of sleep apnoea is Intus Healthcare and the test is called a "Finger Pulse Oximeter Test."

This simple little unit clips gently onto the patients fingertip for one full night's sleep and measures the oxygen saturation levels in their blood through analysing the pulse. The recording is then sent back to the lab for analysis and you will have the results in your hands within 48 hours.

You do NOT need a physician referral for this and I think it cost us around £60 (approximately $95) to have it done.

If you are in any doubt that someone in your care may have sleep apnoea then I strongly advise getting the tests done this way as often waiting for entry into the Sleep Clinics for testing can take precious weeks or even months.

There was some concern now that my father, in his confused state, may not be able to keep the unit on his fingertip overnight, but these concerns proved unwarranted. The care home staff applied the unit to his finger as he fell asleep, and went into his room several times during the night to check it. Come morning it was still attached to him and functioning.

The results quickly came back to the care home, confirming that he displayed the test results showing that he indeed suffered from Mild to Moderate Oxygen Deprivation!

This was another HUGE milestone for us.

I remind you all at this point of Item #3 in the University Research which I outlined in Chapter Ten, which stated, "Putting patients with mild to moderate Alzheimer's on a machine that delivers pressurised air into the lungs during sleep over the course of six weeks resulted in improved test scores for things like verbal learning and mental processing!"

As a sidebar to all of this, I had purchased a second kit so that my Mother could use it on herself at home. This would firstly reassure her how simple it all was and, secondly allay any fears she had that her own mild forgetfulness was anything other than stress related and would be temporary. Her results did indeed come back giving her the all clear.

The next resistance I encountered was that the care home staff understandably felt that my father probably would not tolerate wearing the mask required each night to receive the oxygen. This was only of minimal concern to me. I explained to the physician that I had NOT intended for Dad to wear the mask all night initially!

I truly felt that I did not need my father becoming oxygen dependent by wearing a mask all night every night. I was convinced that even a couple of hours on oxygen each day could make a difference in his cognitive ability and all I was asking was the chance to see if that indeed would prove sufficient.

My first step, once given approval, was to purchase a small fairly inefficient unit for around £60 ($95) and put the mask on Dad while we were visiting him, then, if he tolerated it we could progress to the full unit. This unit (more later) cost me over £900 ($1,200) to purchase, but remember I HAD to buy it as the Doctors would not prescribe it as being necessary. If you present your case using my guidelines you should not have to be faced with this scenario.

The next thing to realise is that your loved one does not have to wear a mask! There is another small nasal applicator which slips gently over the head and inserts in two little prong like tubes slightly into their nostrils and delivers the oxygen. This was taken to readily by my father and most of the time he barely seemed to notice it was in place.

Therefore, knowing that we had proven that he indeed suffered from sleep apnoea and that he could tolerate the nasal applicator, I was now finally ready to bring in the big unit and see if it made a difference!

Suggestion #12

The Patient does NOT have to wear a mask. There is a small tube (nasal applicator) which slips gently over their head and has two little prong like tubes which fit slightly into their nostrils and delivers the oxygen. This is often much more readily acceptable to them. A few days spent using a cheap unit will get the patient used to the nasal applicator before you put out the expenditure of the larger and much more effective unit.

Unless the sleep apnoea is classified as severe, in the initial trial of oxygen the patient does NOT have to keep the oxygen on overnight. We do not want them to become oxygen dependent if at all possible. We simply want to see what difference two hours of oxygen delivery daily will make to them and to document any measurable changes in their behaviours over a period of a few weeks. This is hardly an unreasonable or unsafe request to make of the physician.

Chapter 13

Now I finally felt primed for action in moving my Dads health forward. Thanks to a very knowledgeable and good friend, Richard Swift, in London, I completely changed my approach towards the Medical Consultant.

Firstly, I reminded the consultant that all I was asking for was a trial of oxygen. Then I reminded him of the Hippocratic Oath he had taken of first to do no harm to his patients. In this light he was obligated to try any possible means of help which would be least dangerous. Surely Oxygen must fall into that category?

Secondly, I wrote a separate email and changed my approach from "Can you consider giving my father oxygen?" to "Can you tell me specifically why you are refusing to give my father oxygen?"

This tactical change had an immediate effect. The Consultant responded by saying that he had no objection to me placing my father on a trial of oxygen but that he could not authorise it on a medical prescription for nursing staff to implement as there was insufficient evidence of its effectiveness.

So now I questioned that, apparently now it was acceptable to the physician for my 84 year old, blind in one eye, mother, to apply the oxygen to my father daily, but not acceptable for a trained nurse to do so! The irony of this is inescapable.

(Let me be clear that I am not necessarily being critical of the Consultant personally. He was only responding to the situation according to his training and was allowing me to proceed in the only way he knew how).

Once again thanks to Richard Swift, I had also discovered a company which sold portable oxygen units to the public. These units are about the dimensions of a small suitcase, are easily maneuvered on a wheeled base, simply plug into a wall socket, do not require an oxygen tank, are very simple to operate and are almost noiseless in operation! This solved several problems for me. Firstly the fact that it did not require the use of an oxygen cylinder made it possible to bring it into the care home, as oxygen cylinders require stringent set up requirements and also have different insurance issues for the care home. Secondly it was lightweight and easy to move and would not take up a lot of space in my father's small room. Thirdly it was so simple to operate that my mother could turn it on and off quite easily.

So, finally, by the end of October 2010 we were ready to get Dad started on daily oxygen, however my happiness was tempered with the knowledge that I had been fighting for him since before July 2009 so at least 15 precious months had been lost.

Suggestion #13

It took me over 15 months to get the trial of oxygen approved for my father. Use the tools given in these lessons and you can have it for your loved one in a matter of weeks. Remind the physician of the Hippocratic Oath they took which states "first to do no harm" to their patients and therefore their obligation to try treatments which have least possibility of harming their patients. Oxygen surely must fall into that category. Then make sure you stop asking for a prescription for oxygen and change your approach to asking them why they are refusing to give your loved one a trial of oxygen.

(The company I purchased the unit from for my father was http://bit.ly/portableO2 and the Invacare Unit was the one I purchased although I am sure they will have even more advanced models by the time you read this).

Part 2

Before we move on to the celebrations of signs
of recovery I will supply you with areas other
than oxygen that are worth considering.

Chapter 14

Fire Hazards . . . Fire Doors . . . Evacuation Procedures
should be checked and verified as authentic. Also why the temperature in
the patient's room is so important and what you can do to ensure that it is
kept appropriate and safe for your loved ones.

For these next four chapters I am going to focus on some other issues which well may have relevance for many other families, then I will return to how we applied the oxygen and the many miraculous signs of recovery that we witnessed in my father.

However, first let me address the rooms with closed doors and the high temperatures of the environment.

As my Dad deteriorated he had stopped all walking and did not want to go to the dayroom for any group activities or even to go to the dining room to eat with the other residents. He really wasn't able to communicate sensibly any more. It was the summer of 2010 and prior to the use of oxygen. My mum would visit him each day and they would sit there together in his small room with the temperature rising steadily!

I asked the staff if we could leave his room door open to allow a better flow of air (there was no point in opening the window as the heat wave we were experiencing would only have made things worse). The staff member insisted on keeping his door closed, stating that it was a fire regulation! Now, many years earlier I had been the fire marshal in a general hospital in Canada for a prolonged period and knew that her statement was highly unlikely to be of any value to patient safety. Firstly, if my Father's door was indeed in any way flame retardant it would have to have a solid internal core. A simple rap with your knuckles on a door will let you know if the inside is really solid or not. My Dad's door was almost hollow to knock on and was probably particle board at best and was therefore definitely not a fire door, therefore there was no reason to keep it closed for that purpose.

Some will tell you that it will limit smoke from entering and this is also not true. The smoke and poison fumes from a fire in these facilities usually comes in quickly through the ceilings and is the major cause of loss of life (even when not tiled), so evacuation is the priority NOT keeping the door closed. The ONLY time I would recommend a room's doors be closed is when the fire is in that room. If this EVER happens to you, do NOT try to put out the fire, yell for help first and make sure someone hears you. [It has sadly happened in the past that the one who finds a fire and tries to put it out is very quickly overcome with smoke and then they are unconscious on the floor and still no one else is aware that there is an emergency unfolding and the fire service has not been called.] Next if the fire is anything bigger than a waste basket, get the patient out of the room any way you can and CLOSE THE DOOR. Do Not Try To Put It Out! Never open the door to see how it's doing, you will simply feed the fire oxygen and it will accelerate instantly. Get the patient and yourself out and let the professionals do their job.

Before your loved one is placed in their care, ask the care homes to show you their firewalls and evacuation procedures. Actually my father was initially placed in a room in the floor above ground level rooms and the thought of how these patients would get out in the event of a fire had always been a slight concern to me. We put his name down for a transfer to the ground floor rooms as soon as a vacancy arose and were much happier when this happened.

However, back to the high temperature in my Dad's room.

The staff member still refused to leave my father's door open.

So, first I went out and bought a large (and mostly silent running) fan and placed it on top of his wardrobe in an effort to get air circulating in the tiny room without blowing directly on him and upsetting him. I asked the staff to leave it on day and night. Then I went to the local Garden Centre and bought a thermometer which we hung on a wall in Dads room overnight. When we returned the next day we were stunned to see that the temperature in his room was showing as 92° Fahrenheit (33° Celsius)! I was outraged. My father was sitting in a room in extreme heat all day and all night and no one seemed to care! I asked the staff to turn the temperature setting down on the heating system and was told that there was nothing that could be done as "It's an old heating system and the whole building is at that temperature and there's nothing can be done about it!" So, not only my Dad, but every patient in the facility was enduring this extreme heat and were confused, sleepy and dehydrated (many without even a fan in their room) but everyone seemed to think this was somehow acceptable! This temperature also was affecting the staff as their work areas were no cooler. I ask you now to honestly consider how these high temperatures will cause dehydration in anyone, never mind these already ill and vulnerable patients? Their water intake MUST be increased and monitored as a priority.

This could not continue, so I immediately requested that the staff obtain a letter from the physician in charge of the care home stating that he was aware of the temperature in my father's room and that in his opinion it was safe and acceptable for his patient to be confined in these circumstances!

This seemed to have a positive effect, as, on returning the next day I found that the temperature in my father's room (and indeed the whole facility) was now 70° Fahrenheit (21° Celsius)! I am sure this huge victory alone had been a factor in stopping my father's deterioration and discomfort.

To recap here, what have I fought for so far for my Dad: Oxygen, Water, and a Decent Room Temperature! Basic human survival needs, nothing more, nothing less.

Suggestion #14

Check Evacuation procedures for patients. Check that fire doors really are acceptable grade fire doors. Make sure there is air movement in the patients' rooms, place a fan there yourself if you have to and make sure it stays on day and night if necessary. Monitor the room temperature regularly.

Chapter 15

Many of today's older generation have been exposed to heavy metal toxicity in their work environment which are now proven to lead to many medical disorders. Find out what these are and how to have them safely removed from their systems.

My father's generation were exposed to many heavy metals such as lead, mercury, zinc, aluminium, asbestos, arsenic etc. and a cursory review of today's evidence shows some examples of the effects of these substances such as:

- Aluminium lodged in the brain can cause Alzheimer's.
- Mercury lodged in the brain can cause Autism Spectrum Disorders.
- Iron lodged in the heart tissue can cause heart disease.
- Lead lodged in the bones can interfere with red and even white cell production.

A blood test alone cannot accurately determine the level of metal toxicity in the body. Make sure you request the physician do blood, urine and if agreeable, hair samples for testing.

The most widely accepted treatment for removal of these metals from the body is known as Chelation Therapy and its effectiveness is now widely accepted in conventional and complimentary medical circles.

Chelation therapy involves your doctor or naturopath placing an IV line into the arm (or other location), then dripping a chelation agent into your bloodstream. The most common chelation agent used today is ethylenediaminetetraacetic acid or EDTA. As the University of Maryland Medical Center explains, "Chelation therapy using EDTA is the medically accepted treatment for lead poisoning. . . . Other heavy metal poisonings treated with chelation include mercury, arsenic, aluminum, chromium, cobalt, manganese, nickel, selenium, zinc, tin, and thallium. Chelating agents other than EDTA are also used to clear several of these substances from the bloodstream."

This page goes on to explain, "Heavy metal toxicity in humans has been associated with many health conditions, including heart disease, attention deficit/hyperactivity disorder(ADHD), Alzheimer's disease, immune system disorders(including irritable bowel syndrome, or IBS), and autism." [http://bit.ly/EDTAmmc]

Learn more: "How to test for metals poisoning and remove heavy metals from your body" [http://bit.ly/mtlspoison]

I have been given further opinion that fluoride in the water may be connected to the metals binding down in the brain. You may not be able to eliminate fluoride from your local water supply but please take whatever steps you can to get it filtered in your homes, work places and care home environments.

I knew that my father had been exposed to high levels of asbestos over the years and also had many mercury fillings in his teeth. I asked for the tests to be performed on my father, but, as far as I recall, they never happened. Ask yourself how many cases of dementia could be stopped or reversed by early implementation of these tests and procedures?

Suggestion #15

In the early stages of dementia insist if you have to that the physician perform the appropriate tests for the presence of Heavy Metals in the body and then, if found that chelation therapy or equivalent be implemented, then retest for Metals.

Chapter 16

Benefits of early intervention by using Hyperbaric Chambers are explained and also by early onset screening to determine possible traumatic and reversible damage to the brain by an advanced Myofascial or Cranio Sacral Therapist. On another note, there are many claims now that coconut oil often produces a dramatic improvement in people with dementia/Alzheimer's. I suggest that you research that for yourself.

I have now shown that when the early signs of dementia are identified that tests for sleep apnoea and also a check for Heavy Metals should be an automatic and standard check, and that, if either test is positive, chelation therapy and oxygen therapy should be implemented immediately. There is precedent for this form of treatment in other illnesses. For example, Autistic children are being successfully treated in centres known as Autism One Centres with a regime which includes Chelation Therapy and Oxygen Saturation by placing them in a Hyperbaric Chamber for short spells.

In the early stages of forgetfulness there would be no difficulty in getting the patient to accept the Hyperbaric Chamber as a possible solution.

Patients with other illnesses such as Parkinson's disease have also been medically prescribed similar treatments in Hyperbaric Chambers, so for you to request this could not be considered unreasonable. If the physician says there is insufficient proof that it works, refer to the evidence I have provided earlier and remind him/her that it is not contraindicated therefore how, in all conscience, can they deny you the right to try?

There is yet another area which is not considered in early identification and treatment of Alzheimer's/dementia and that is any history of head injury.

My father had three falls throughout his life that I know of and struck the back of his head in each instance. Just as severe blows to the head can cause brain damage to an athlete or a fighter in the ring then there is the feasible possibility that falls could also cause lasting damage in one way or another.

Apart from bruising and chronic swelling around the brain there is another little known system that could well be contributing. This system is known as Myofascia or Connective Tissue. It is a dense web-like substance that surrounds every muscle, ligament, joint and organ in the human body. In the relaxed state it transfers nutrition and information to and from every cell in the human body. However, under stress, such as an impact injury, it goes into a frozen, protective state to protect the body.

I have studied all facets of this system and am qualified as an Advanced Myofascial Therapist so I am well placed to speak on this topic. The only way to see if possible restrictions are there and can be eliminated is by being examined by an Advanced Myofascial Therapist or an Advanced Cranio-Sacral Therapist. Two or Three treatments will determine if there is any noticeable change in the patient's dementia or Alzheimer's symptoms.

Suggestion #16

In the early stages of dementia, have the patient assessed and treated by an Advanced Myofascial Therapist or Cranio-Sacral Therapist for two or three treatments to see if there are noticeable positive changes.

For more information on this feel free to contact me at my website: http://kineticchainrelease.com or on Facebook at Kinetic Chain Release: https://www.facebook.com/KCR11.

On another note there appears to be growing evidence that Coconut Oil has been responsible for some spectacular improvements in dementia/Alzheimer's disease. I am unable to comment further but suggest that you research it for yourself.

Chapter 17

Another simple example of how dementia patients can lose mobility in care home scenarios, and yet another simple fix.

There is one other simple thing to watch out for on behalf of your loved ones in institutional care. That is the tables sometimes used to place their meals/snacks on when they are unable to leave their bedside chair. These tables often have a frame on wheels at the bottom which allows staff to put the tray section close in for the patient to eat from. The bar at the bottom of this can often be seen at worst to almost pin the patients legs against the chair and, at least to prevent them from straightening their legs. Try sitting like this for a few hours every day and then try to get up and walk! They can't straighten their legs! Then family are told that Mum or Dad can't walk as well. This is NOT the staff's fault. It is simply an improvement which needs to be implemented now. All they have to do is lift the patient's feet and place them on the other side of the base bar. This problem can disappear overnight!

Suggestion #17

Make sure that the food table at the bedside chair does not restrict the ability of the patient to straighten his or her legs if they want to.

Part 3

Let the party begin! My family AND the medical staff in the care home began to work together and excitedly witness and document the incredible changes in my father's condition as he regained more and more mental acuity and physical capabilities. Then we PROVE that the symptoms of dementia/Alzheimer's are indeed reversible!

Chapter 18

We finally bring O₂ to my father and begin his journey of reconnection with reality.

So, finally, by the end of October 2010 we were ready to get Dad started on daily oxygen, however my happiness was tempered with the knowledge that I had been fighting for him since before July 2009 so at least 15 precious months had been lost.

I had purchased a unit, known as a Portable Oxygen Delivery Unit. It cost me around £900 but the cost was not important to me and I gladly bore the cost myself. (this is not an attempt at grandstanding on my part . . . this is to reaffirm that when action needs to be taken, understandably not all medical or even family members will be fully in agreement . . . the only important thing is to simply get on with it). The company I purchased the unit from can be seen at http://bit.ly/portableO2 and the unit I purchased was very similar to the Invacare Perfecto 2 model.

It is quiet and compact. It electronically separates oxygen from the air in the room and delivers it to the patient at whatever flow rate it is set at.

Remember, and I cannot repeat this often enough, I did NOT want my Dad put on Oxygen all night every night. (for this they use a unit known as a CPAP unit). I felt this could make him oxygen dependent. I simply wanted him on Oxygen for 2 hours each day and then note if we noticed any significant physical or cognitive changes.

It really was a very simple and logical request.

So we finally brought the unit into Dad's room. I showed the care home administrator how it operated, to ensure that she was satisfied that it met all safety standards for her institution. Then showed all the staff, nurses and carers, so they knew what it was and what it was to be used for.

As I had been given no input from the physician, I had to decide what setting to use for my father. Thankfully my years of working in High Dependency Units (I.C.U.) gave me enough knowledge to proceed safely. I set the initial dosage at a flow of 2.5 litres per minute, and when no adverse effects were noted after three weeks, I increased the flow to 3.0 litres per minute. The amount of time the unit was used each day sadly varied tremendously, anywhere from 20 minutes per day to three hours per day, depending on how long my mother could be there. There were also several days when she could not get there as the weather was too severe and other times when she was ill with the flu etc. and had to miss a few days visiting. She would be absolutely distraught at the thought of not seeing Dad and the fact that he wasn't receiving his oxygen and we often had to calm her as best we could, and to remind her that, without her efforts, Dad would have been receiving any oxygen at all.

How much easier and consistent it all would have been if the care home nursing staff had been allowed to simply switch the machine on and off and document it. We'll never know how much further forward my Dad would have come with this medical cooperation in place, but, as you will come to see, the chances that his improvements would have been faster, sustained and improved upon are very probable indeed.

However, what had long seemed impossible to me was now happening. My Dad was receiving oxygen to see if it affected the symptoms of Alzheimer's disease!

Suggestion #18

Make In the last resort, if you meet a lot of resistance from the care home or physician, remind them that you could bring your loved one food, drink, cigarettes, alcohol or drugs and they (the staff) would never know or even ask! Then tell them that you are bringing a safe oxygen unit in on a certain date and let them try to justify stopping you. Use this book to get staff cooperation from the beginning so that the oxygen can be applied consistently and easily for an agreed period of time. I suggest a six weeks trial period.

Chapter 19

Within 3 weeks the miracles begin to unfold and then the medical profession gradually begins to come on board!

Within 3 weeks of oxygen delivery to my Dad, as outlined in the previous chapter, we, the family, and the care home staff began to notice MANY positive changes in his behaviours and interactions, which continued over the next 3 months!

Miracle: We suddenly noticed that he was once again referring to his childhood home when he interacted with us. He had not done this for quite a few months!

Miracle: He began to talk of his mother again on occasion, something we had also not heard for some time!

Miracle: Staff had noted and then documented how he was communicating better with them and was much more cooperative!

Miracle: Next he began to talk about his days in the Royal Navy during World War II and where he had been stationed and his involvement with the midget submarine unit, and of his wartime experience in the Shetland Islands!

Miracle: Then, unprompted by us he began recalling his father's occupation and also reminisced over the three dogs he had owned as a young boy and as a young man!

All small things in themselves but when put together it was as though he was coming back up through the layers of confusion to levels we had not seen in close to a year!

Miracle: He actually began to hold small, but intelligent conversations periodically, something noted by family and staff alike!

Miracle: He frequently, although not always, recognized his sons again, which was so satisfying for us when we saw the light of recognition in his eye!

Now, these itemised episodes may not seem like a lot to those who have not gone through the Alzheimer's experience with a loved one, however we, like other families (and care staff) were in no way prepared for my father actually reversing the downward spiral and returning back to a level we hadn't seen for months! We were truly excited and, just to see him improve, even for a minute was a sheer delight and something that often sustained us for days! The Miracles were indeed unfolding.

Miracle: We got our first big breakthrough in cooperation from the medical world!

Such was the impressive level of improvement noted by staff and family, and reported to the Physician, that the Physician (GP) called a meeting in mid December 2010 (less than 2 months from oxygen being administered) with the G.P., my family, a nurse practitioner and a staff nurse from the care home in attendance. The staff nurse was in concurrence with our family that there were marked improvements in Dad's behaviours on many levels, noted not just by our family, but by several members of care support staff who worked with my father daily.

Based on the consistency of the evidence provided, coupled with the fact that the improvements had sustained for several months and that ongoing improvement was still apparent to all: The physician, obviously impressed, eagerly agreed to write to the Consultant to request a medical prescription for Oxygen treatment for my father. If approved, this would mean that nursing staff could administer it daily and consistently in a structured format, and improvements could be more accurately identified and documented.

The Consultant quickly responded that, based on the evidence provided, he now had no objection to my father being given Oxygen on a medical referral and left the final decision back with the G.P.

We had come such a long way from feeling like a voice in the wilderness in the world, to amazingly now having the full written support of the consultant, the physician, nursing staff, support staff and care home administration to administer oxygen to my father. Now the urgency intensified for us to continue the progress made so far.

Suggestion #19

Once Oxygen begins to be given daily, make certain that you document any and all changes noted in the patient's behaviours or capabilities. Make certain that all staff are also documenting anything noteworthy. These changes will seem small and almost insignificant at first but quickly will form together to show a sustained improvement which will clearly manifest as an indisputable gradual reversal of symptoms.

Chapter 20

The current tests to show mental improvement in patients with Alzheimer's appear to be totally inadequate and inappropriate.

The staff were also instructed by the physician to give my father the standard tests to verify cognitive improvements. A good idea in principle, however, these tests are grossly inadequate and their format does not demonstrate any true values or indicators in these cases where the dementia is already well advanced. These tests ask questions like "What day of the week, or date, is it today?" and "Who is the Prime Minister?"

These patients have no idea what day of the week it is. To them every day is Groundhog Day, their routine never varies, they awaken, eat, sleep at the same times, and over 90% of their conversations are the same as the day before! Even the staff admitted they sometimes have trouble remembering which day it is!

I feel, that for the more advanced Alzheimer's patients that care staff and family are best positioned to notice, validate and document improvements, as they are the ones in most constant interaction with the patient, and are familiar with their recent and long term awareness and levels of understanding.

So, in conclusion. The standard cognitive tests should be used while the dementia is manifesting initially, however, by the time the patient requires full time care these tests are totally inadequate as a measure of improvement or deterioration.

Once again I remind you of how revolutionary my approach was and is to the medical system. They HAVE NO TESTS in place to measure improvement in dementia patients, BECAUSE THEY HAVE NO CONCEPT THAT THIS COULD BE A POSSIBILITY . . . until my Dad showed up on the radar!

Suggestion #20

Sit with care home staff in weekly meetings if possible and discuss and document changes noted in the patient. It will be totally different for every patient as their severity and indeed their life experiences will have been entirely different.

Chapter 21

The saddest chapter of all. The medical system reduced my father's oxygen supply drastically and "coincidentally" he began to deteriorate rapidly. I cannot and would not say categorically that this was in any way intentional or was a factor in his death but it does leave many questions unanswered, particularly in the light of the next two joyous chapters.

I want to deliver the saddest chapter now as I want you to end this book in total celebration with me, and you will! However, along with the good news we were hit with yet another unexpected delay and ultimately I suspect and truly feel was a fatal blow to my father and to our efforts. The G.P. insisted on Pulmonary Function tests being carried out before approval would be given! This, in spite of the fact that my father had been on Oxygen for nearly 4 months almost daily with no adverse effects noticed or documented! We had no choice but to comply. My father was finally taken to hospital for the authorized testing over a month later on the 30th of March 2011, and it was an incredible 8 weeks later (almost 2 months) on the 25th of May 2011 that my father was given a medical referral to have daily oxygen as a viable treatment for the symptoms of dementia. The physician then delivered another body blow to us and indeed allowed the nurses to apply oxygen although only at a rate of 1 litres flow per minute, which was 2 litres less than Dad had been receiving!. The physician said that if Dad showed no ill effects after a few weeks then he could be retested for pulmonary function and levels of 2 litres per minute implemented. This would still not have returned him to the 3 litres he had been thriving on prior to medical intervention. We were not allowed to deliver oxygen at the former rate.

Again after 2 months of no ill effects (yet beginning to clearly deteriorate mentally) Dad was again sent to the hospital for more tests and waited over two months, again, for the results. We never did get even the 2 litre flow implemented. During this time, after amazing changes had happened until the oxygen was cut back, Dad had rapidly deteriorated mentally and physically and on October 9th 2011 he quietly passed away.

In essence, by approving oxygen and placing blocks on its implementation my father was denied further progress for months and after this 5 months of steady deterioration he passed away.

I rage at the incompetencies in the medical system which, in my mind and heart, are clearly culpable here. When you read the next joyous chapter you will rage also and I urge you not to tolerate this nonsense on any level should you be faced with a similar scenario in the future.

Suggestion #21

1. To wait for over a month on two separate occasions to have my father given simple pulmonary function tests is an indictment of the NHS in the UK and is totally unacceptable.

2. To have to wait over 2 months on both occasions to receive the results of these tests is beyond irresponsible and borders on medical negligence.

3. For the physician to, in effect, deny my father the use of oxygen at a level he had been receiving, is, in my opinion, at the least illogical and at worst incompetent and negligent.

4. I would have overridden the physician and returned Dad to 3 litres per minute daily, but the machine was now set with an alarm which would notify nursing staff if the pre-set low flow was adjusted so we were in essence being denied that chance to assist Dad in any way. Do NOT allow this to happen.

5. Do NOT accept any decrease in oxygen flow for your loved ones. Use this story as your leverage. Get a lawyer if you have to. Stand your ground.

6. If Pulmonary Function tests need to be done, get them done privately. It will be money well spent, I promise you.

7. If you think it may not be worth the effort, wait until you read the next chapter!

When you absorb this upcoming chapter of just how far he came before being restricted you will be overjoyed and impressed beyond belief. I thank God that we all got the opportunity to share these amazing times with him and now thank God that I can share them with you.

Chapter 22

The first delay of almost 3 months in getting approval for oxygen for my father proved to be a true blessing in disguise, as, during that time we could still give him two hours of oxygen at a flow of 3 litres per minute daily, and it is in that three month window when he showed the most stunning and incredible improvements! Let me list some of them for you now.

Miracle: My father had deteriorated to such a level that when we asked him what time it was he would just look at us blankly. If we asked where was his watch or the wall clock in front of him he would get confused and not relate at all. One day, without being prompted, he suddenly said "It's 4:30 exactly" and it was! He then began to tell my mother what a beautiful watch he had and how it kept remarkably accurate time indeed! The staff were quickly brought in so he could tell them too! Our shock and then our joy was boundless! Please take a moment now to imagine how that must have felt.

Miracle: A staff member couldn't wait to tell us her experience with my Dad. Apparently she came in to take him for a bath. She hadn't been on that particular shift for a few weeks so hadn't seen him at bath time for a while. She chatted away to him as she always would have and told him she would just take his watch off and leave it in his bedroom so she wouldn't mistakenly leave it in the bathroom. She said he raised an eyebrow and said "Not like you did the last time you took me for a bath!" She said she almost literally fell over when he said that, as she had indeed forgotten his watch the last time she had taken him, which was several weeks prior! She almost tearfully ran to tell all of the other staff and to document the conversation, and couldn't wait to tell my mother the following day.

Miracle: One day, at the end of visiting hours Mum gave him her usual kiss goodbye and we shook his hand. As Ma got to the door, he pursed his lips showing her he wanted a kiss. She told him she already gave him one. He shook his head and looked dejected. Mum sighed and walked back to him and planted another kiss on his lips. As she straightened up, his face broke into the biggest grin and he gave me the two thumbs up sign! He had just conned her into another kiss! We laughed long and hard over this one.

Miracle: On occasion, Dad would still allow staff to wheel him into the activity room, but really had stopped almost all forms of interaction while there. One activity had the person in charge throwing a soft rubber ball to patients, who were supposed to catch it and throw it back. Dad just let it bounce off of him. One day he suddenly headed the ball back, soccer style, right to the staff member and called out "Do it again!" The staff member obliged and Dad would sometimes return the ball accurately with a header or even on occasion kicked it back from seated in his wheelchair! [When my father was the young man he was very athletic and in fact was being scouted for professional soccer before World War II appeared and he enlisted in the Royal Navy.] The staff member in charge of activities was also clearly excited and affected by Dad's recovery and couldn't wait to tell other staff, family and to document.

Miracle: Dad enjoyed when the local Christian group showed up. He didn't care what denomination they were, he just wanted to join in the Hymn singing. It was so heartening for us all to sit with him, listen to him and see how much he was enjoying himself.

Miracle: He started walking again!! From being a patient who had great difficulty sometimes even with help to be transferred from his wheelchair to his bed, he began to walk for increasing distances down the hallway with his Zimmer Frame walker. I made sure that staff saw me take him for those walks and they began to encourage him also.

Miracle: As I said earlier dad had pretty much become resident in his room, he had stopped going down to the dining room at all and was eating very sparsely for the most part. He suddenly became abundantly cooperative and had returned to being in the dining room for all three meals each day, sometimes walking down and back!

Miracle: My Dad was the king of one liner jokes, often a man of few words but with a laser like sense of humour. He began suddenly throwing these *zingers* into seemingly unrelated conversations and very much kept us all on our toes at times. He would literally have us in tears laughing at him.

Miracle: One day, Mum couldn't get in to see him, so she called the care home to inform him. They decided to put Dad on the phone to her and they had a dialogue where he clearly understood why she couldn't come, and that she would see him the following day. They had not had a telephone conversation in over three years!

Miracle: Dad went out on short trips with other residents in the community wheelchair accessible bus! This at least got him out seeing life, traffic and places he hadn't seen in a long time. He seemed to en-joy these trips if they didn't overload him on a sensory level. Care must be taken when taking patients out into the world if they haven't been exposed to it for a while. It needs to be in short spells at first, gradually expanding their horizons. However, we were just delighted that he was participating.

Now, put all of these things together over a two month period and how do you feel about it all? You can only begin to imagine how we and the care home staff felt, while Dad was clearly enjoying the interactions also. And the two biggest *miracles* of all were yet to come!

Suggestion #22

Believe in Miracles and you WILL witness them. Then be prepared to stand your ground and create even more, in places where traditional medicine has failed to create any.

Chapter 23

On Saturday July 9th 2011, the biggest miracle of all!
My father walked up his own driveway again and
visited with his family again for two hours!

Despite some mental deterioration, which I firmly believe was due to having oxygen delivery greatly reduced, Dad continued to walk with his walker frame and hold conversations at times and, **on Saturday July 9th 2011, the biggest and happiest miracle of all. My father walked up his own driveway again and returned to visit his home for two hours!** I ask you now, how many Alzheimer's Patients do you know that have gone as far down the rabbit hole of confusion as my father had gone only to return somehow to a state where they could revisit their home?

He was helped out of the minibus and stood looking at his home for a minute or two, before, using his Zimmer Frame walker, beginning to walk down the pathway to his front door. My Mother stood on the path, tears in her eyes, as she watched her beloved begin to walk towards her. I was just behind him in case he should falter, which he never did and my wife Jane was beside him. He suddenly stopped, looked around for a moment, then turning to Jane he looked her in the eyes and said "I can handle this." Then, halfway down the path, he stopped and pointed to the large garbage bins and said to Jane, "Those were mine!" "They went out front!" He had always put the bins out onto the sidewalk (pavement) weekly for collection for many years. So he did indeed know where he was! This totally amazed and stunned us, yet it scared us in some unspoken ways as we wondered what else he remembered and if indeed was more aware of the helplessness of the surroundings in the care home than we had realised! We will never know the answer for sure to that question.

There are three quite steep steps into my parent's home and Dad would have had difficulty negotiating them so going inside and seeing what else he recalled was not an option.

It was a beautiful summer's day, not a breath of wind, flowers in full bloom and Mum had set up a table and chairs outside on the back patio. Dad walked all the way to behind the house unassisted and sat down as directed, with Mum at his side. For the next two hours they were together again, having tea and Dad holding various levels of conversations with Mum, Jane, my brother John and me. To say it was wonderful, to say it was unbelievable, to say it was emotional does not begin to clarify how we all felt, including Dad, who was very much at peace, alert and interactive throughout the time. Many a quiet tear was shed by all at different times throughout this family gathering as it unfolded.

Suggestion #23

From January 2009 when my father was admitted to a care home, incontinent and incoherent and was clearly dying before our eyes, to him not only surviving for a further two and a half years but actually reversing the Alzheimer's deterioration and coming back home for a visit in July 2011 was beyond any of our wildest dreams and the memories we hold of this and other interactions are a great source of comfort to us now, and should be a beacon for millions of other families.

Our joy was tempered with sadness when the visit came to an end. The miracle came with a price to pay. The care home staff came to pick Dad up again and he seemed confused then his eyes filled with tears when he realised they were taking him away again! What a terrible heart wrenching moment that proved for us all. I went back with him to the care home

And, as I pushed his wheelchair back into the entrance area his eyes filled with tears yet again! I whispered to him that it was OK and that he would be going back regularly once a week for a wee visit and that was something he could look forward to. He nodded and squeezed my hand. With a huge lump in my throat I watched the staff wheel him back to his room, wondering if we had done the right thing even beginning oxygen, Would it not have been better to leave him in his demented unknowing state and avoid this pain? If he indeed had begun to visit weekly it would have become more accepted I am sure. There was never any notion entertained by any of us that Dad may someday actually return home to live. He still required full-time nursing care, but to enjoy a weekly visit for a couple of hours for a cup of tea and a chat could well have become an enjoyable part of the interactions.

However, due mostly to inclement weather, he never did get the chance to return home and it was 3 months to the day when he finally passed away. However I reiterate that the memories of that blessed day of celebration that he came home has sustained me and most of us through many a dark time since his passing.

Chapter 24

One last miracle.

Dad presented himself to the world as we all remembered him, one last time.

One final miracle. Dad fluctuated back and forth during the next few weeks and, when offered to go out on a day trip with other residents, happily complied although anything beyond three hours seemed like over stimulation to him and he would become increasingly uncomfortable and confused, then loud and occasionally angry with all around him as he wanted to return to the familiarity of his room, but again I stress for 2 hours or so he was generally perfectly behaved and cooperative. He had not had outdoor social interaction with the family as a whole since July 9th, however on September 21st my Mums older brother was celebrating his 90th birthday in a local hotel/restaurant and Dad gladly agreed to attend, looking very much like his old self in a white shirt and his blue Royal Navy tie, his navy blue jacket and his grey flannel, impeccably creased trousers and polished shoes, hair and nails neatly trimmed and tidy. He came in a wheelchair and did not walk at this event, he had in essence begun to deteriorate physically, but he sat there, 91 years young, along with his 87 year old sweetheart, his 90 year old brother-in-law and Jane, along with our dear friends John and Shiela Freil, and everyone thoroughly enjoyed the occasion. They began an impromptu sing along together along with another family who were seated nearby (who were also celebrating a 90th birthday for one of their members) which caused great interest from people at other tables until a full blown sing along was in effect! The hotel staff even joined in the fun, although when the waiter took orders from those present for more coffee or tea, he omitted to ask my father. Dad called him back and, raising one eyebrow in the way only Dad could, firmly told him he had been omitted and ordered another cup of coffee for himself! He returned to the care home afterwards in excellent frame of mind and happy with the stimulation of the day's events. I could not attend that particular event, but I am not sorry I didn't see it personally. I simply revelled then and revel now in the delicious knowing that he DID it!

Once more I ask you to picture and FEEL the happiness and joy of all of these events from a family perspective and then to reflect on how NONE of the changes and joy mentioned in the last few chapters would have happened if he had not received oxygen!

Suggestion #24

Once you have achieved the "impossible" and have given the patient access to increased social stimuli to which they clearly enjoy, it is imperative that you must continue the process, no matter what it may take to do so. You can NOT let them experience it then take it away again. That is not acceptable.

Ensure their oxygen intake remains high and their external stimulus of family events and interactions remains constant for as long as you can.

Part 4

I bring our story to an end and pass
the torch of hope to all of you.

Chapter 25

Throughout this journey, as my Dad showed improvement after improvement, I contacted Alzheimer's Scotland and Europe, repeatedly offering the tangible proof of what I was claiming, which was that Oxygen delivery can at a minimum slow and at best reverse the body, mind and soul numbing process of Alzheimer's disease. I asked them to publish it in their newsletters and periodicals to at least stimulate conversation and awareness. They refused, stating that they didn't want to give people false hope! I was absolutely stunned to hear this. How dare they deny people ANY hope in a world where all medications have proven useless in slowing the disease yet are increasingly prescribed to our loved ones, with never a thought as to how these meds interact or the slightest thought that progress is an option to consider.

I responded with these 2 emails:

Subject: Leo Gilbert

Today My 91 year old Dad Came Home to his house for 2 HOURS! the first time in 2.5 years! (for those who haven't followed this saga, he has Alzheimer's) The amazing thing was he clearly REMEMBERED where he was and was SOOO happy. This alone stimulated him to conversations of a whole new level.

My Mother was in tears of happiness. When it came time to go back to the care home his eyes filled with tears although he kept his head high. My brother stood quietly watching with a tear in his eye also. My partner, Jane has shed many a tear today also. I sat with Dad when he was back in the care home until he could come to terms with it and he knows he can go back, hopefully, 2 or 3 times a week, depending on Mum's health.

So Please don't tell me that Oxygen does not help dementia, the changes have been astounding, and please Alzheimer's Scotland don't tell me again that you won't publish this story as you don't want to give people false hope . . . firstly we have NO hope under the current care plan, it is simply a long goodbye, so ANY hope and ANY signs of improvement are welcomed with open hearts, no matter how transient they may prove to be . . . and secondly what about the difference O_2 has made to my father's quality of life . . . doesn't that matter . . . ?

He is walking up to 8 meters again at a time, is eating 3 full meals a day again, and is able to return to his HOME again and sit in his own garden . . . please share this story,

Namaste,

Hugh

Subject: Leo Gilbert

I resend my previous correspondence as an attachment, plus I now add the fact that Dad came out to a function in a hotel just 2 weeks ago and was able to converse with guests and waiters etc. (all things we could never have dreamed of before) should give an indisputable mountain of anecdotal and research material . . . added of course to the many other articles now supporting O_2 deficiency (and H_2O deficiency as potential prime factors in dementia).

Best Wishes,

Hugh Gilbert

As I write this now, two years to the day since my father passed, to the best of my knowledge, Alzheimer's Scotland and Alzheimer's Europe remain silent.

Chapter 26

We end our journey together (for now).

It seems that nothing has changed. Just today I read the media hype about a new wonder drug which will help eliminate Alzheimer's. Many people I know are excited about this "breakthrough." However, when I took the time to read the whole article, two things became clear. Firstly the "wonder drug" works on the plaque cells in the brain, which they still stubbornly believe are the cause of Alzheimer's disease.

Having read this book you now understand the extremely high probability that these cells are formed due to a chronic lack of oxygen to the brain . . . therefore they are directing the "wonder drug" at a symptom and not addressing the probable cause.

Secondly, they go on to state that they hope to have the drug in production within the next 10 years! Not really a lot to celebrate there is there. The bullshit continues.

I have offered you as many insights as possible in this story that it may give you more than hope and instil a determination to prevent others from suffering the potentially unnecessary indignities and insults of the horrors of Alzheimer's disease.

I remain available for further discussion or general contact at my email of **yahugh@journeysend.ca**

or my websites:

http://hughgilbert5D.com
http://kineticchainrelease.com

If I can help in any way do not hesitate to get in touch.

Wishing you all peace of mind body and spirit and praying that this book may just make a difference,

Love and Gratitude,

Hugh

List of Suggestions

Suggestion #1

"You have an obligation to protect the caregiver (in this case my Mum) just as much as to protect and support the loved one suffering from Alzheimer's."

The one who is caring for the other is on a slippery slope to a breakdown in their health as well. They are caring for a loved one in often almost intolerable circumstances as the dementia increases. The constant worry and stress of dealing with the complete unpredictability of their loved ones behaviour takes an unavoidable toll. Do NOT listen to them when they stoically tell you that they are coping well. Either step in to help them yourself or get professional assistance involved in day to day care immediately. In retrospect I wish we had taken this step a long time before the end game kicked off.

Suggestion #2

When you have a relative beginning to show early signs of any form of dementia, have the foresight to find what care home facilities are available locally for if and when the time should come.

Ask for a full tour of each of them and be clear as to what level of care each provides and what are the admission criteria. Families don't do this because they feel guilty and because they are still in denial that it won't become necessary.

We could have, and on reflection should have, gone around these care homes at least a year prior to being confronted with the necessity. We could have done this without telling or upsetting my mother and thus been much better prepared to deal with it.

Suggestion #3

Moving Dad created a lot of hurt internally in our family, as I'm sure it has in millions of others. Things were said in the chaos of the moment that left scars for some time to come. On reflection none of it was meant as negative or intended to hurt, but was simply an understandable response to the insanity we were all being forced to deal with. Please, please realise that stress affects each family member differently and they will process their grief differently, and sometimes even wear rose tinted glasses of denial—the first stage of grieving. Do not try to get everyone feeling the same or to take anything they may say personally. It will only create even more pain and stress if you do. Everyone recognise each other's right to be confused and afraid and simply be as compassionate as you can while remembering to be gentle on yourself too!

Suggestion #4

To all readers, if you see a loved one deteriorate rapidly in similar circumstances, please ensure that their fluid intake is closely monitored and that they are being given adequate and timely assistance to reach the toilet when they need it. Please also insist that if they are deteriorating that they may well be dehydrated and could be rehydrated by means of a saline drip intravenously where possible, as recovery of mental alertness due to this simple intervention can often be instant and seemingly miraculous.

Suggestion #5

My Questions regarding sleep apnoea:

"Could this 40 years of nightly O_2 (oxygen) deprivation to the brain be a contributing factor to the aberrant changes in cellular struc-ture and diminishment in size of the brains of dementia/Alzheimer's sufferers?"

If so, then, "Could an increase in that oxygen supply give some return of physical and mental capability and function to my Dad and in fact to the millions of other dementia/Alzheimer's sufferers globally?"

And, beyond that, "If my first question was true, then could oxygen possibly be used as a preventative measure for the millions of others showing early signs of dementia?"

Suggestion #6

When your loved ones become agitated do not simply dismiss it as their being delusional, they may well be having an experience beyond our comprehension, and it is just as terrifying for them as it would be for us.

Support them as best you can until they are calm again. It wouldn't hurt to establish if there has been a history of paranormal activity in the building or in their room before.

I know this may sound a little off the wall to some of you, but I can only relate it as it happened and give the best advice accordingly.

Suggestion #7

If your parent, living at home, eventually requires home care assistance, make certain that a family member is at hand every day for the first few days until your parent becomes comfortable with the individual(s) and the process.

Suggestion #8

When a parent is initially placed in a care home facility, often it is the one who has taken care of the finances throughout their marriage. The remaining parent is initially totally bewildered by the apparent complexity of handling ongoing bills etc. and has much worry as to how future income (pensions etc.) will be impacted by their current situation. Therefore it is imperative that family are aware of this and quietly set about taking care of some of the bills by paying for the basics until everything has settled into a routine again. In our case, to ease the transition, as stated, we paid for Mum's phone bill, her Television billings and for 2 years we paid for the carer who eventually was employed to come into her home twice a week for 2 hours each time. Each family should find their own ways of providing such support and discuss it well in advance of the need arising.

This may not be necessary at all but should be prepared for and once implemented can take two to three years before no longer being necessary.

Suggestion #9

When you have a relative in a care home scenario please understand that, to staff there, the thought that a patient in their care may actually improve is almost beyond their comprehension initially. This has never happened to any of their patients in the past and is understandably a completely foreign and illogical concept for them. Be prepared to use this story as a means of education as it will be vital for you to get them on board as quickly as possible. If your loved one is still at home it should be much easier to pursue.

Suggestion #10

This article was published in the *Red Deer Advocate* newspaper (Red Deer, Alberta, Canada) on Oct. 1st 2009 by Lee Bowman and was discussing a publication in the medical journal, Diabetes Care.

This is powerfully important information for families who are trying to get access to oxygen to help their loved ones.

1. "Some studies show that as many as 70% to 80% of all dementia patients also suffer from sleep apnoea!"

2. "Scientists at The University of San Diego, California, last year for the first time showed that treating sleep apnoea in patients with Alzheimer's actually seemed to improve cognitive function"

3. "Specifically, putting patients with mild to moderate Alzheimer's on a machine that delivers pressurised air into the lungs during sleep over the course of six weeks resulted in improved test scores for things like verbal learning and mental processing!"

4. "A Study by the University of Washington School of Medicine found that chronic sleep deprivation makes the brain plaques that characterise Alzheimer's disease appear earlier and more often."

Please pay FULL attention to this last statement. It is compelling evidence of the proof you have been looking for.

Suggestion #11

The U.K. Company who provided the kit to test my father for a diagnosis of sleep apnoea is Intus Healthcare and the test is called a "Finger Pulse Oximeter Test."

This simple little unit clips gently onto the patients fingertip for one full night's sleep and measures the oxygen saturation levels in their blood through analysing the pulse. The recording is then sent back to the lab for analysis and you will have the results in your hands within 48 hours.

You do NOT need a physician referral for this and I think it cost us around £60 (approximately $95) to have it done.

Suggestion #12

The Patient does NOT have to wear a mask. There is a small tube (nasal applicator) which slips gently over their head and has two little prong like tubes which fit slightly into their nostrils and delivers the oxygen. This is often much more readily acceptable to them. A few days spent using a cheap unit will get the patient used to the nasal applicator before you put out the expenditure of the larger and much more effective unit.

Unless the sleep apnoea is classified as severe, in the initial trial of oxygen the patient does NOT have to keep the oxygen on overnight. We do not want them to become oxygen dependent if at all possible. We simply want to see what difference two hours of oxygen delivery daily will make to them and to document any measurable changes in their behaviours over a period of a few weeks. This is hardly an unreasonable or unsafe request to make of the physician.

Suggestion #13

It took me over 15 months to get the trial of oxygen approved for my father. Use the tools given in these lessons and you can have it for your loved one in a matter of weeks. Remind the physician of the Hippocratic Oath they took which states "first to do no harm" to their patients and therefore their obligation to try treatments which have least possibility of harming their patients. Oxygen surely must fall into

85

that category. Then make sure you stop asking for a prescription for oxygen and change your approach to asking them why they are refusing to give your loved one a trial of oxygen.

Suggestion #14

Check Evacuation procedures for patients. Check that fire doors really are acceptable grade fire doors. Make sure there is air movement in the patients' rooms, place a fan there yourself if you have to and make sure it stays on day and night if necessary. Monitor the room temperature regularly.

Suggestion #15

In the early stages of dementia insist if you have to that the physician perform the appropriate tests for the presence of Heavy Metals in the body and then, if found that chelation therapy or equivalent be implemented, then retest for Metals.

Suggestion #16

In the early stages of dementia, have the patient assessed and treated by an Advanced Myofascial Therapist or Cranio-Sacral Therapist for two or three treatments to see if there are noticeable positive changes.

Suggestion #17

Make sure that the food table at the bedside chair does not restrict the ability of the patient to straighten his or her legs if they want to.

Suggestion #18

Make In the last resort, if you meet a lot of resistance from the care home or physician, remind them that you could bring your loved one food, drink, cigarettes, alcohol or drugs and they (the staff) would never know or even ask! Then tell them that you are bringing a safe oxygen unit in on a certain date and let them try to justify stopping you. Use this book to get staff cooperation from the beginning so that the oxygen can be applied consistently and easily for an agreed period of time. I suggest a six weeks trial period.

Suggestion #19

Once Oxygen begins to be given daily, make certain that you document any and all changes noted in the patient's behaviours or capabilities. Make certain that all staff are also documenting anything noteworthy. These changes will seem small and almost insignificant at first but quickly will form together to show a sustained improvement which will clearly manifest as an indisputable gradual reversal of symptoms.

Suggestion #20

Sit with care home staff in weekly meetings if possible and discuss and document changes noted in the patient. It will be totally different for every patient as their severity and indeed their life experiences will have been entirely different.

Suggestion #21

1. To wait for over a month on two separate occasions to have my father given simple pulmonary function tests is an indictment of the NHS in the UK and is totally unacceptable.

2. To have to wait over 2 months, on both occasions, to receive the results of these tests is beyond irresponsible and borders on medical negligence.

3. For the physician to, in effect, deny my father the use of oxygen at a level he had been receiving, is, in my opinion, at the least illogical and at worst incompetent and negligent.

4. I would have overridden the physician and returned Dad to 3 li-tres per minute daily, but the machine was now set with an alarm which would notify nursing staff if the pre-set low flow was adjusted so we were in essence being denied that chance to assist Dad in any way. Do NOT allow this to happen.

5. Do NOT accept any decrease in oxygen flow for your loved ones. Use this story as your leverage. Get a lawyer if you have to. Stand your ground.

6. If Pulmonary Function tests need to be done, get them done privately. It will be money well spent, I promise you.

7. If you think it may not be worth the effort, wait until you read the next chapter!

Suggestion #22

Believe in Miracles and you WILL witness them. Then be prepared to stand your ground and create even more, in places where traditional medicine has failed to create any.

Suggestion #23

From January 2009 when my father was admitted to a care home, in-continent and incoherent and was clearly dying before our eyes, to him not only surviving for a further two and a half years but actually reversing the Alzheimer's deterioration and coming back home for a visit in July 2011 was beyond any of our wildest dreams and the memories we hold of this and other interactions are a great source of comfort to us now, and should be a beacon for millions of other families.

Suggestion #24

Once you have achieved the "impossible" and have given the patient access to increased social stimuli to which they clearly enjoy, it is imperative that you must continue the process, no matter what it may take to do so. You can NOT let them experience it then take it away again. That is not acceptable.

Ensure their oxygen intake remains high and their external stimulus of family events and interactions remains constant for as long as you can.

Author Profile

Hugh Gilbert is a Physical Therapist, Published Author, International Speaker and Lecturer educated initially in Glasgow, Scotland and after 35 years in Canada has returned to teach in the U.K. while still teaching throughout North America and has taught in Mexico, Argentina and Hawai'i. Hugh is also a Registered Independent Medical Consultant and Advanced Myofascial Therapist. His amazing protocol "Kinetic Chain Release" is his Intellectual Property and has been accepted for Continuing Education Credits by The Scottish Massage Therapy Association; The Irish Physical Therapy Association; The Missouri Physical Therapy Association; The Canadian Sports Massage Therapists Association; The Arizona School of Integrated Studies; and The Alberta Association of Massage Therapists. Hugh was a keynote speaker at the World Conference of Complementary Medicine in Santa Fe and has been an assistant instructor at the Presentation of Myofascial Release to the American Back Society Conference in Orlando. During this time, Hugh gained extensive insights over the years as a trusted consultant to industry and insurance companies. Over the last 3 decades, he has maintained balance in his education in other ways, much of his interest directed towards not only industry but also sports, culminating in five years as Head Coach at University level in Canada He is grateful for the invaluable experience gained by involvement in other areas such as the Skate Canada Championships and the Canadian National Basketball Championships.

In other areas, Hugh has been an ongoing student of and now a recognized International Teacher of Energy Work; Hawaiian Healing Studies; Celtic Healing; Native American Studies; is an Ordained Minister of Spiritual Peacemaking, and has presented Interfaith Workshops. He has successfully implemented conflict resolution strategies for families and corporations.. Much of Hugh's recent work has evolved around success working with Autistic and Attention Deficit children, their parents, teachers and caregivers.

For more information on Alzheimer's or any other areas of interest please contact Hugh at:

www.kineticchainrelease.com
www.hughgilbertauthor.com
www.hughgilbert5D.com
or email at **yahugh@journeysend.ca**

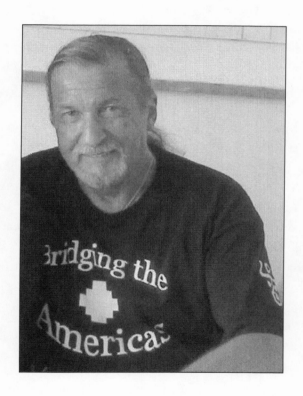

Made in the USA
Charleston, SC
17 October 2014